The Ultimate Vegetarian Savory Recipe Book

Tasty And Easy Savory Vegetarian Dishes

Adam Denton

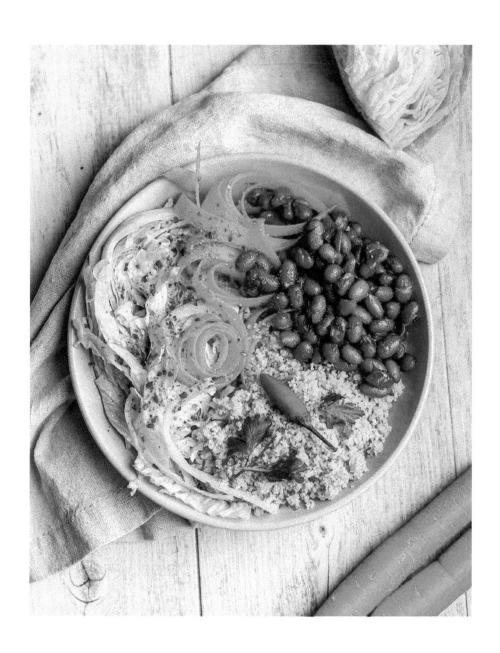

Table of contents

Farfalle Pasta in Spicy Chimichurri Sauce with Ricotta

Ingredients

5 jalapeno peppers

1 yellow onion, chopped

15 ounce can butterbeans, rinsed and drained

15 ounce can borlotti beans , rinsed and drained

4 tbsp. chimichurri sauce

1/2 tsp. cayenne pepper

½ teaspoon salt

1/8 teaspoon black pepper

2 cups vegetable stock

8 ounces farfalle pasta uncooked

1 ½ cups Ricotta Cheese

Garnishing ingredients:

chopped green onions for serving

Directions:

Put all of the ingredients except for pasta, vegan cheese, and garnishing ingredients in your slow cooker. Combine and cover. Cook on high heat for 4 hours or low heat for 7 hours. Add the pasta and cooking on high heat for 18 minutes, or until pasta

becomes al dente Add 1 cup of cheese and stir. Sprinkle with the remaining cheese and garnishing ingredients Elbow

Spaghetti with Green Olives and Tomatoes

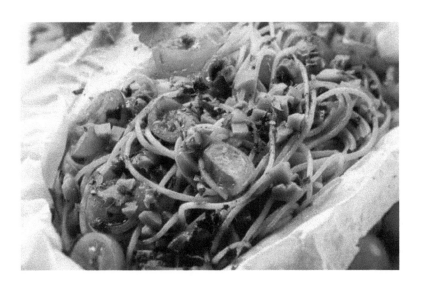

Ingredients

1 red onion, medium chopped

1 green bell pepper chopped

28 ounce crushed tomatoes

1/4 cup green olives

2 tbsp. capers

½ teaspoon salt

1/8 teaspoon black pepper

2 cups vegetable stock

8 ounces spaghetti noodles uncooked

1 ½ cups Vegan Cheese (Tofu Based)

<u>Garnishing ingredients:</u>

chopped green onions for serving

Directions:

Put all of the ingredients except for pasta, vegan cheese, and garnishing ingredients in your slow cooker. Combine and cover. Cook on high heat for 4 hours or low heat for 7 hours. Add the pasta and cooking on high heat for 18 minutes, or until pasta becomes al dente Add 1 cup of cheese and stir. Sprinkle with the remaining vegan cheese and garnishing ingredients.

Penne Pasta with Chorizo and Pecorino Romano

Ingredients

1 red onion, medium chopped

28 ounce crushed tomatoes

1/4 cup vegan chorizos, coarsely chopped

1 tsp. dried thyme

½ teaspoon salt

1/8 teaspoon black pepper

2 cups vegetable stock

8 ounces penne pasta uncooked

½ cup Pecorino Romano Cheese

½ cup Mozarella cheese

½ cup cheddar cheese

Garnishing Ingredients:

chopped green onions for serving

Directions:

Put all of the ingredients except for pasta, vegan cheese, and garnishing ingredients in your slow cooker. Combine and cover. Cook on high heat for 4 hours or low heat for 7 hours. Add the

pasta and cooking on high heat for 18 minutes, or until pasta becomes al dente Add 1/2 cup of mozzarella cheese & ½ cup of cheddar cheese and stir. Sprinkle with the remaining pecorino romano cheese and garnishing ingredients

Slow Cooked Fettuccini with Mozarella

Ingredients

1 red onion, medium chopped

1 green bell pepper chopped

15 ounce sour cream

28 ounce crushed tomatoes

2 tbsp. tomato paste

1 tsp. basil

1 tsp. Italian seasoning

½ teaspoon salt

1/8 teaspoon black pepper

2 cups vegetable stock

8 ounces fettuccini uncooked

1 ½ cups Mozarella Cheese (Tofu Based)

Garnishing Ingredients:

chopped green onions for serving

Directions:

Put all of the ingredients except for pasta, vegan cheese, and garnishing ingredients in your slow cooker. Combine and cover. Cook on high heat for 4 hours or low heat for 7 hours. Add the

pasta and cooking on high heat for 18 minutes, or until pasta becomes al dente Add 1 cup of mozzarella cheese and stir. Sprinkle with the remaining cheese and garnishing ingredients

Farfalle Pasta with Ricotta Cheese

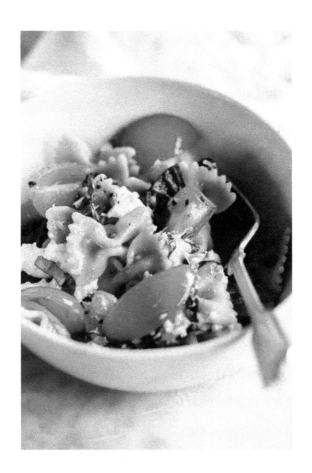

Ingredients

1 yellow onion, medium chopped

1 red bell pepper, chopped

28 ounce canned green tomatoes

1/4 cup green olives

2 tbsp. capers

½ teaspoon salt

1/8 teaspoon black pepper

2 cups vegetable stock

8 ounces farfalle pasta uncooked

1 ½ cups Ricotta Cheese

<u>Garnishing Ingredients:</u>
chopped green onions for serving

Directions:

Put all of the ingredients except for pasta, vegan cheese, and garnishing ingredients in your slow cooker. Combine and cover. Cook on high heat for 4 hours or low heat for 7 hours. Add the pasta and cooking on high heat for 18 minutes, or until pasta becomes al dente Add 1 cup of cheese and stir. Sprinkle with the remaining ricotta cheese and garnishing ingredients

Spicy Macaroni and Mozarella Cheese

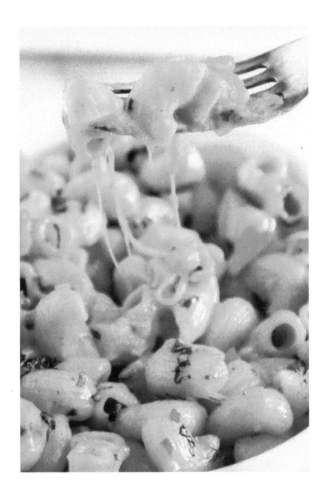

Ingredients

¼ cup extra virgin olive oil

1 red onion

28 ounce crushed tomatoes

½ teaspoon salt

1/8 teaspoon black pepper

2 cups vegetable stock

8 ounces whole wheat elbow macaroni pasta uncooked

1 ¼ cups Mozarella Cheese (Tofu Based)

¼ cup Parmigiano Regiano Cheese

Garnishing Ingredients:

chopped green onions for serving

Directions:

Put all of the ingredients except for pasta, vegan cheese, and garnishing ingredients in your slow cooker. Combine and cover. Cook on high heat for 4 hours or low heat for 7 hours. Add the pasta and cooking on high heat for 18 minutes, or until pasta becomes al dente Add 1 cup of cheese and stir. Sprinkle with the remaining vegan cheese and garnishing ingredients

Pappardelle Pasta with Mozarella Cheese

Ingredients

1 red onion, medium chopped

15 ounce can lima beans, rinsed and drained

15 ounce can borlotti beans , rinsed and drained

28 ounce crushed tomatoes

4 tbsp. cream cheese

1 tsp. herbs de Provence

½ teaspoon salt

1/8 teaspoon black pepper

2 cups vegetable stock

8 ounces pappardelle pasta uncooked

1 ½ cups mozarella Cheese

<u>Garnishing Ingredients:</u>

chopped green onions for serving

Directions:

Put all of the ingredients except for pasta, vegan cheese, and garnishing ingredients in your slow cooker. Combine and cover. Cook on high heat for 4 hours or low heat for 7 hours. Add the pasta and cooking on high heat for 18 minutes, or until pasta

becomes al dente Add 1 cup of mozzarella cheese and stir. Sprinkle with the remaining cream cheese, mozzarella cheese and garnishing ingredients

Pasta Shells with Chimichurri Sauce and Gouda Cheese

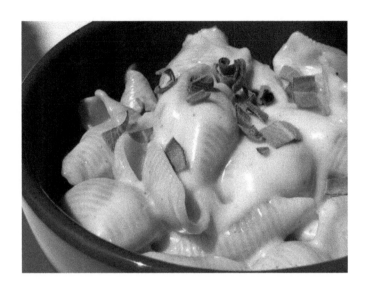

Ingredients

1 red onion, medium chopped

5 jalapeno peppers

1 red onion

4 tbsp. chimichurri sauce

1/2 tsp. cayenne pepper

½ teaspoon salt

1/8 teaspoon black pepper

2 cups vegetable stock

8 ounces pasta shells uncooked

1 ½ cups gouda cheese (Tofu Based)

Garnishing Ingredients:

chopped green onions for serving

Directions:

Put all of the ingredients except for pasta, vegan cheese, and garnishing ingredients in your slow cooker. Combine and cover. Cook on high heat for 4 hours or low heat for 7 hours. Add the pasta and cooking on high heat for 18 minutes, or until pasta becomes al dente Add 1 cup of cheese and stir. Sprinkle with the remaining cheese and garnishing ingredients

Penne Pasta with Mozarella and Gorgonzola Cheese

Ingredients

1 red onion, medium chopped

28 ounce crushed tomatoes

3 ounces vegan mozzarella

1 tsp. Italian seasoning

½ teaspoon salt

1/8 teaspoon black pepper

2 cups vegetable stock

8 ounces penne pasta uncooked

1 ½ cups mozzarella Cheese

¼ cup Gorgonzola cheese

Garnishing Ingredients:

chopped green onions for serving

Directions:

Put all of the ingredients except for pasta, vegan cheese, and garnishing ingredients in your slow cooker. Combine and cover. Cook on high heat for 4 hours or low heat for 7 hours. Add the pasta and cooking on high heat for 18 minutes, or until pasta

becomes al dente Add 1 cup of cheese and stir. Sprinkle with the remaining vegan cheese and garnishing ingredients.

Spaghetti with Kalamata Olives

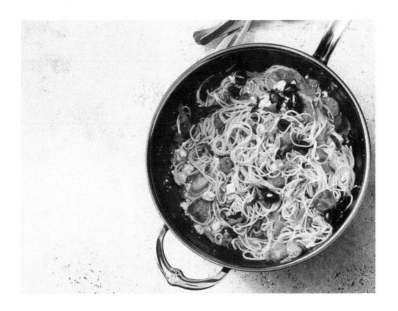

Ingredients

1 red onion, medium chopped

¼ cup kalamata olives

28 ounce crushed tomatoes

4 tbsp. pesto

1 tsp. Italian seasoning

½ teaspoon salt

1/8 teaspoon black pepper

2 cups vegetable stock

8 ounces spaghetti noodles uncooked

1 ½ cups Vegan Cheese (Tofu Based)

Garnishing Ingredients:

chopped green onions for serving

Directions:

Put all of the ingredients except for pasta, vegan cheese, and garnishing ingredients in your slow cooker. Combine and cover. Cook on high heat for 4 hours or low heat for 7 hours. Add the pasta and cooking on high heat for 18 minutes, or until pasta becomes al dente Add 1 cup of cheese and stir. Sprinkle with the remaining cheese and garnishing ingredients

Elbow Macaroni with Vegan Chorizo and Green Olives

Ingredients

1 red onion, medium chopped

1 green bell pepper chopped

½ cup green olives, drained

9 cloves garlic, minced

28 ounce crushed tomatoes

1/4 cup vegan chorizos, coarsely chopped

1 tsp. dried thyme

½ teaspoon salt

1/8 teaspoon black pepper

2 cups vegetable stock

8 ounces whole wheat elbow macaroni pasta uncooked

1 ½ cups Mozzarella Cheese

Garnishing Ingredients:

chopped green onions for serving

Directions:

Put all of the ingredients except for pasta, vegan cheese, and garnishing ingredients in your slow cooker. Combine and cover.

Cook on high heat for 4 hours or low heat for 7 hours. Add the pasta and cooking on high heat for 18 minutes, or until pasta becomes al dente Add 1 cup of cheese and stir. Sprinkle with the remaining mozarella cheese and garnishing ingredients.

Penne Pasta with Olives and Cream Cheese

Ingredients

1 red onion, medium chopped

1 green bell pepper chopped

¼ cup olives, drained

¼ cup capers, drained

28 ounce crushed tomatoes

4 tbsp. cream cheese

1 tsp. herbs de Provence

½ teaspoon salt

1/8 teaspoon black pepper

2 cups vegetable stock

8 ounces penne pasta uncooked

1 ½ cups mozzarella cheese

Garnishing Ingredients:

chopped green onions for serving

Directions:

Put all of the ingredients except for pasta, vegan cheese, and garnishing ingredients in your slow cooker. Combine and cover.

Cook on high heat for 4 hours or low heat for 7 hours. Add the pasta and cooking on high heat for 18 minutes, or until pasta becomes al dente Add 1 cup of cheese and stir. Sprinkle with the remaining vegan cheese and garnishing ingredients

Farfalle Pasta with Mozzarella and Capers

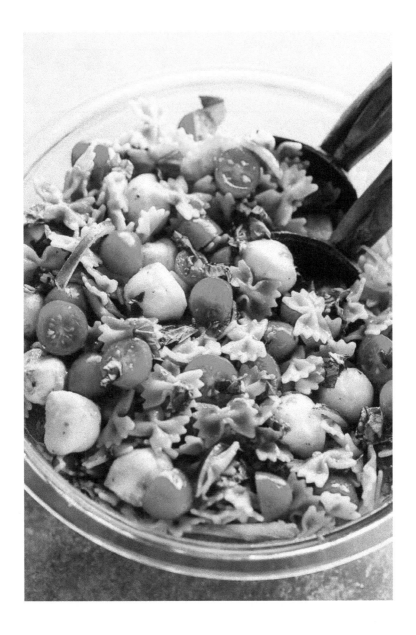

Ingredients

1 yellow onion, medium chopped

¼ cup capers, drained

28 ounce crushed tomatoes

3 ounces vegan mozzarella

1 tsp. Italian seasoning

½ teaspoon salt

1/8 teaspoon black pepper

2 cups vegetable stock

8 ounces farfalle pasta uncooked

1 ½ cups Vegan Cheese (Tofu Based)

Garnishing Ingredients:

chopped green onions for serving

Directions:

Put all of the ingredients except for pasta, cheese, and garnishing ingredients in your slow cooker. Combine and cover. Cook on high heat for 4 hours or low heat for 7 hours. Add the pasta and cooking on high heat for 18 minutes, or until pasta becomes al dente Add 1 cup of cheese and stir. Sprinkle with the remaining vegan cheese and garnishing ingredients

Spaghetti with Oyster Mushrooms

Ingredients

1 red onion, medium chopped

¼ cup oyster mushrooms

15 ounce tomato sauce

28 ounce crushed tomatoes

2 tbsp. tomato paste

1 tsp. basil

1 tsp. Italian seasoning

½ teaspoon salt

1/8 teaspoon black pepper

2 cups vegetable stock

8 ounces spaghetti noodles uncooked

1 ½ cups Vegan Cheese (Tofu Based)

<u>Garnishing Ingredients:</u>

chopped green onions for serving

Directions:

Put all of the ingredients except for pasta, cheese, and garnishing ingredients in your slow cooker. Combine and cover. Cook on high heat for 4 hours or low heat for 7 hours. Add the pasta and cooking on high heat for 18 minutes, or until pasta becomes al dente Add 1 cup of cheese and stir. Sprinkle with the remaining vegan cheese and garnishing ingredients

Penne Pasta with Green Tomatoes in Chimichurri Sauce

Ingredients

1 red onion, medium chopped

1/4 cup vegan Italian sausage, coarsely chopped

1 cup green tomatoes chopped

¼ cup capers, drained

4 tbsp. chimichurri sauce

1/2 tsp. cayenne pepper

½ teaspoon salt

1/8 teaspoon black pepper

2 cups vegetable stock

8 ounces penne pasta uncooked

1 ½ cups Vegan Cheese (Tofu Based)

Garnishing Ingredients:

chopped green onions for serving

Directions:

Put all of the ingredients except for pasta, vegan cheese, and garnishing ingredients in your slow cooker. Combine and cover. Cook on high heat for 4 hours or low heat for 7 hours. Add the

pasta and cooking on high heat for 18 minutes, or until pasta becomes al dente Add 1 cup of cheese and stir. Sprinkle with the remaining vegan cheese and garnishing ingredients

Farfalle Pasta with Vegan Cream Cheese Tomato Sauce

Ingredients

1 yellow onion, medium chopped

1 green bell pepper, chopped

8 ounces, vegan cream cheese

15 ounce tomato sauce

28 ounce crushed tomatoes

1/4 cup green olives

2 tbsp. capers

½ teaspoon salt

1/8 teaspoon black pepper

2 cups vegetable stock

8 ounces farfalle pasta uncooked

1 ½ cups Vegan Cheese (Tofu Based)

Garnishing Ingredients:

chopped green onions for serving

Directions:

Put all of the ingredients except for pasta, vegan cheese, and garnishing ingredients in your slow cooker. Combine and cover.

Cook on high heat for 4 hours or low heat for 7 hours. Add the pasta and cooking on high heat for 18 minutes, or until pasta becomes al dente Add 1 cup of cheese and stir. Sprinkle with the remaining vegan cheese and garnishing ingredients

Elbow Macaroni with Mozzarella and Gorgonzola Cheese

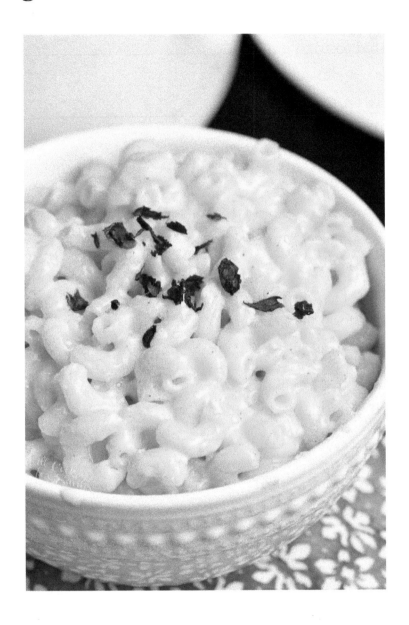

Ingredients

1 red onion, medium chopped

1/4 cup vegan Italian sausage, coarsely chopped

¼ cup red pesto

15 ounce can tomato sauce

28 ounce crushed tomatoes

2 tbsp. tomato paste

1 tsp. basil

1 tsp. Italian seasoning

½ teaspoon salt

1/8 teaspoon black pepper

2 cups vegetable stock

8 ounces whole wheat elbow macaroni pasta uncooked

1 ½ cups Mozarella Cheese

¼ cup gorgonzola cheese

Garnishing Ingredients:
chopped green onions for serving

Directions:

Put all of the ingredients except for pasta, vegan cheese, and garnishing ingredients in your slow cooker. Combine and cover. Cook on high heat for 4 hours or low heat for 7 hours. Add the pasta and cooking on high heat for 18 minutes, or until pasta

becomes al dente Add 1 cup of cheese and stir. Sprinkle with the remaining vegan cheese and garnishing ingredients

Penne Pasta with Capers and Vegan Chorizo

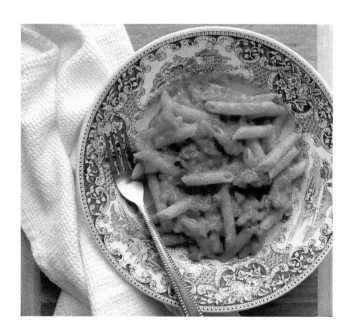

Ingredients

1 ancho chili

1 tsp. Tabasco hot sauce

1 red onion

15 ounce can tomato sauce

¼ cup capers, drained

28 ounce crushed tomatoes

1/4 cup vegan chorizos, coarsely chopped

1 tsp. dried thyme

½ teaspoon salt

1/8 teaspoon black pepper

2 cups vegetable stock

8 ounces penne pasta uncooked

1 ½ cups Mozarella Cheese (Tofu Based)

Garnishing Ingredients:

chopped green onions for serving

Directions:

Put all of the ingredients except for pasta, vegan cheese, and garnishing ingredients in your slow cooker. Combine and cover. Cook on high heat for 4 hours or low heat for 7 hours. Add the pasta and cooking on high heat for 18 minutes, or until pasta becomes al dente Add 1 cup of cheese and stir. Sprinkle with the remaining cheese and garnishing ingredients

Vegetarian Bolognese

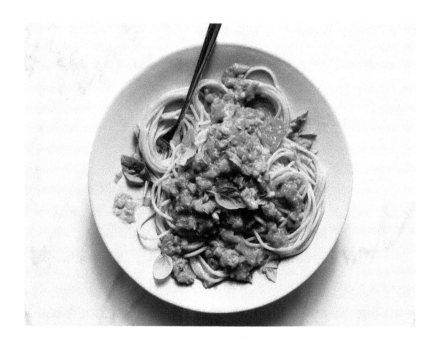

Ingredients

1 large sweet red onion, diced

2 carrots, diced 3 celery stalks, diced 1

2 garlic cloves, minced Sea Salt Black pepper

1 16-ounce bag borlotti beans, rinsed and picked through

2 28-ounce cans crushed tomatoes 5 cups vegetable broth

1 bay leaf

2 tablespoons dried basil

2 teaspoons dried parsley

1 teaspoon coarse sea salt

1/2 – 1 teaspoon crushed red pepper flakes

Directions:

Combine the onion, carrot, celery and garlic thoroughly and season with salt and pepper. Add in the remaining ingredients and stir thoroughly Cook on low for 4 and a half hours, or until lentils begin to soften and sauce becomes thick. Adjust seasoning by adding more salt & pepper to taste.

Red Bean Burrito Bowl with Chimichurri Sauce

Ingredients

1 ancho chili, diced

1 red onion, diced

1 mild red chili, finely chopped

1 1/2 cup red beans

1 cup uncooked white rice

1 1/2 cups chopped tomatoes

1/2 cup water

4 tbsp. chimichurri sauce

1/2 tsp. cayenne pepper

Sea salt

Black pepper

Toppings:

fresh coriander (cilantro), chopped spring onions, sliced avocado, guacamole, etc.

Directions:

Combine all the burrito bowl ingredients (not toppings) in a slow cooker. Cook on low for 3 hours, or until the rice is cooked. Serve hot with topping ingredients

Black Rice Burrito Bowl with Vegan Chorizos

Ingredients

5 Serrano peppers, diced

1 red onion, diced

1 mild red chili, finely chopped

1 1/2 cup navy beans, drained

1 cup uncooked black rice

1 1/2 cup chopped green tomatoes

1/2 cup water

1/4 cup vegan chorizos, coarsely chopped

1 tsp. dried thyme

Sea salt

Black pepper

Toppings:

fresh coriander (cilantro), chopped spring onions, sliced avocado, guacamole, etc.

Directions:

Combine all the burrito bowl ingredients (not toppings) in a slow cooker. Cook on low for 3 hours, or until the rice is cooked. Serve hot with topping ingredients

Vegetarian Chimichurri Burrito Bowl

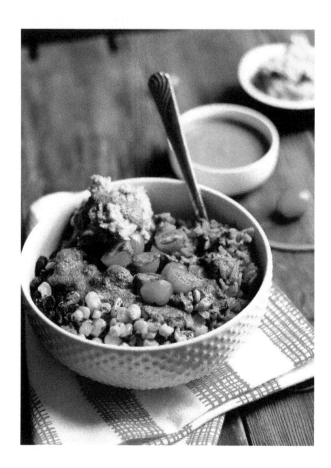

Ingredients

1 red onion, diced or thinly sliced

1 green bell pepper (I used yellow), diced

1 mild red chili, finely chopped

1 ½ cups black beans, drained

1 cup Vegan Italian sausage, coarsely chopped

1 cup uncooked brown rice

1 ½ cups chopped tomatoes

½ cup water

4 tbsp. chimichurri sauce

1/2 tsp. cayenne pepper

Sea salt

Black pepper

Toppings:

fresh coriander (cilantro), chopped spring onions, sliced avocado, guacamole, etc.

Directions:

Combine all the burrito bowl ingredients (not toppings) in a slow cooker. Cook on low for 3 hours, or until the rice is cooked. Serve hot with topping ingredients

Vegetarian Black Rice Burrito Bowl

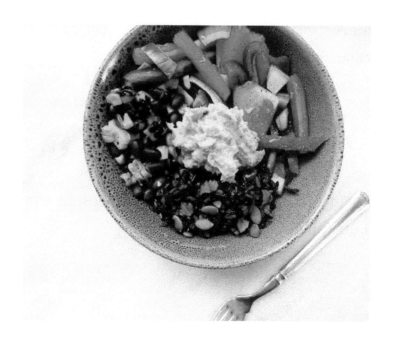

Ingredients

1 poblano chili, diced

1 red onion, diced

1 mild red chili, finely chopped

1 1/2 cup navy beans, drained

1 cup uncooked black rice

1 1/2 cup chopped green tomatoes

1/2 cup water

8 tbsp. pesto

1 tsp. Italian seasoning

Sea salt

Black pepper

<u>Toppings:</u>

fresh coriander (cilantro), chopped spring onions, sliced avocado, guacamole, etc.

Directions:

Combine all the burrito bowl ingredients (not toppings) in a slow cooker. Cook on low for 3 hours, or until the rice is cooked. Serve hot with topping ingredients

Brown Rice with Vegetarian Sausage and Black Bean Burrito Bowl

Ingredients

5 jalapeno peppers, diced

1 red onion, diced

1 mild red chili, finely chopped

1 ½ cups black beans, drained

1 cup uncooked brown rice

1 ½ cups chopped tomatoes

½ cup water

1/4 cup vegetarian grain meat sausage (brand: Field Roast), coarsely chopped

1 tsp. dried thyme

Sea salt

Black pepper

Toppings:

fresh coriander (cilantro), chopped spring onions, sliced avocado, guacamole, etc.

Directions:

Combine all the burrito bowl ingredients (not toppings) in a slow cooker. Cook on low for 3 hours, or until the rice is cooked. Serve hot with topping ingredients

Black Rice with Vegan Italian Sausage

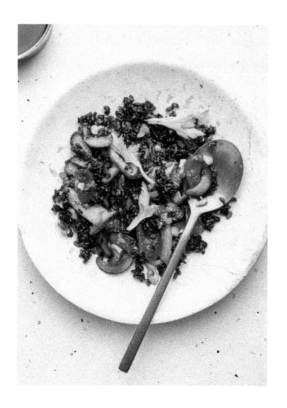

Ingredients

1 red onion, diced or thinly sliced

1 green bell pepper (I used yellow), diced

1 mild red chili, finely chopped

1 1/2 cup vegan Italian sausage, crumbled

1 cup uncooked black rice

1 1/2 cup chopped tomatoes

1/2 cup water

1/4 cup vegan chorizos, coarsely chopped

1 tsp. dried thyme

Sea salt

Black pepper

Toppings:

fresh coriander (cilantro), chopped spring onions, sliced avocado, guacamole, etc.

Directions:

Combine all the burrito bowl ingredients (not toppings) in a slow cooker. Cook on low for 3 hours, or until the rice is cooked. Serve hot with topping ingredients

Brown Rice and Vegan Meatballs

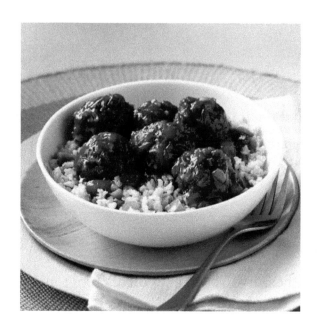

Ingredients

1 Anaheim pepper, diced

1 red onion, diced

1 mild red chili, finely chopped

1/2 cup meatless meatballs, crumbled

1 cup uncooked brown rice

1 ½ cups chopped tomatoes

½ cup water

4 tbsp. vegan cream cheese, sliced thinly

1 tsp. herbs de Provence

Sea salt

Black pepper

<u>Toppings:</u>

fresh coriander (cilantro), chopped spring onions, sliced avocado, guacamole, etc.

Directions:

Combine all the burrito bowl ingredients (not toppings) in a slow cooker. Cook on low for 3 hours, or until the rice is cooked. Serve hot with topping ingredients

Chipotle Black Rice Burrito Bowl

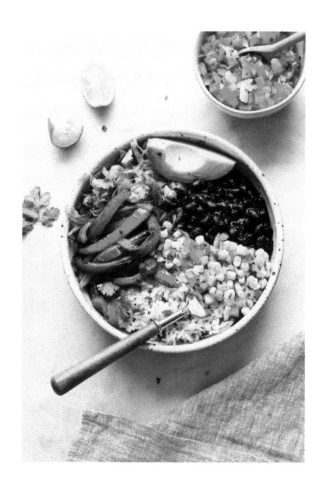

Ingredients

5 Serrano peppers, diced

1 red onion, diced

1 mild red chili, finely chopped

1 1/2 cup navy beans, drained

1 cup uncooked black rice

1 1/2 cup chopped tomatoes

1/2 cup water

1 tbsp chipotle hot sauce (or other favorite hot sauce)

1 tsp smoked paprika

1/2 tsp ground cumin

Sea salt

Black pepper

Toppings:

fresh coriander (cilantro), chopped spring onions, sliced avocado, guacamole, etc.

Directions:

Combine all the burrito bowl ingredients (not toppings) in a slow cooker. Cook on low for 3 hours, or until the rice is cooked. Serve hot with topping ingredients

Pesto Brown Rice Burrito Bowl

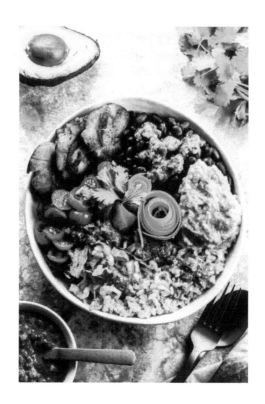

Ingredients

5 jalapeno peppers, diced

1 red onion, diced

1 mild red chili, finely chopped

1 ½ cups black beans, drained

1 cup uncooked brown rice

1 ½ cups chopped tomatoes

½ cup water

4 tbsp. pesto

1 tsp. Italian seasoning

Sea salt

Black pepper

Toppings:

fresh coriander (cilantro), chopped spring onions, sliced avocado, guacamole, etc.

Directions:

Combine all the burrito bowl ingredients (not toppings) in a slow cooker. Cook on low for 3 hours, or until the rice is cooked. Serve hot with topping ingredients

Black Rice and Vegan Sausage Burrito Bowl

Ingredients

1 red onion, diced or thinly sliced

1 green bell pepper (I used yellow), diced

1 mild red chili, finely chopped

1/2 cup vegetarian grain meat sausages, crumbled

1 cup uncooked black rice

1 1/2 cup chopped tomatoes

1/2 cup water

4 tbsp. vegan cream cheese, sliced thinly

1 tsp. herbs de Provence

Sea salt

Black pepper

Toppings:

fresh coriander (cilantro), chopped spring onions, sliced avocado, guacamole, etc.

Directions:

Combine all the burrito bowl ingredients (not toppings) in a slow cooker. Cook on low for 3 hours, or until the rice is cooked. Serve hot with topping ingredients

Spicy Brown Rice Burrito Bowl with Cream Cheese

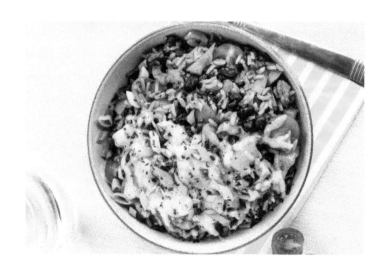

Ingredients

5 Serrano, diced

1 red onion, diced

1 mild red chili, finely chopped

1/2 cup vegan burger (Brand: Beyond Meat Beyond Burger), crumbled

1 cup uncooked brown rice

1 ½ cups chopped tomatoes

½ cup water

4 tbsp. vegan cream cheese, sliced thinly

1 tsp. herbs de Provence

Sea salt

Black pepper

<u>Toppings:</u>

fresh coriander (cilantro), chopped spring onions, sliced avocado, guacamole, etc.

Directions:

Combine all the burrito bowl ingredients (not toppings) in a slow cooker. Cook on low for 3 hours, or until the rice is cooked. Serve hot with topping ingredients

Black Rice with Pesto and Anaheim Peppers

Ingredients

1 Anaheim pepper, diced

1 red onion, diced

1 mild red chili, finely chopped

1 1/2 cup fava beans, drained

1 cup uncooked black rice

1 1/2 cup chopped tomatoes

1/2 cup water

4 tbsp. pesto

1 tsp. Italian seasoning

Sea salt

Black pepper

Toppings:
fresh coriander (cilantro), chopped spring onions, sliced avocado, guacamole, etc.

Directions:

Combine all the burrito bowl ingredients (not toppings) in a slow cooker. Cook on low for 3 hours, or until the rice is cooked. Serve hot with topping ingredients

Brown Rice and Black Beans with Capers

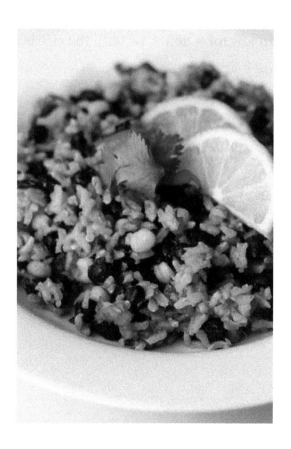

Ingredients

5 jalapeno peppers, diced

1 red onion, diced

1 mild red chili, finely chopped

1 ½ cups black beans, drained

1 cup uncooked brown rice

1 ½ cups chopped tomatoes

½ cup water

4 tbsp. cream cheese, sliced thinly

¼ cup capers, drained

Sea salt

Black pepper

Toppings:

fresh coriander (cilantro), chopped spring onions, sliced avocado, guacamole, etc.

Directions:

Combine all the burrito bowl ingredients (not toppings) in a slow cooker. Cook on low for 3 hours, or until the rice is cooked. Serve hot with topping ingredients

Black Rice with Vegan Chorizo & Olives

Ingredients

1 ancho chili, diced

1 red onion, diced

1 mild red chili, finely chopped

¼ cup capers, drained

¼ cup olives, drained

1 cup uncooked black rice

1/2 cup vegan burger (Brand: Beyond Meat Beyond Burger), crumbled (optional)

1/2 cup vegan Chorizo (Soyrizo), crumbled (optional)

1 1/2 cup chopped tomatoes

1/2 cup water

1 tbsp chipotle hot sauce (or other favorite hot sauce)

1 tsp smoked paprika

1/2 tsp ground cumin

Sea salt

Black pepper

Toppings:
fresh coriander (cilantro), chopped spring onions, sliced avocado, guacamole, etc.

Directions:

Combine all the burrito bowl ingredients (not toppings) in a slow cooker. Cook on low for 3 hours, or until the rice is cooked. Serve hot with topping ingredients

Spicy Vegan Chorizo Chili

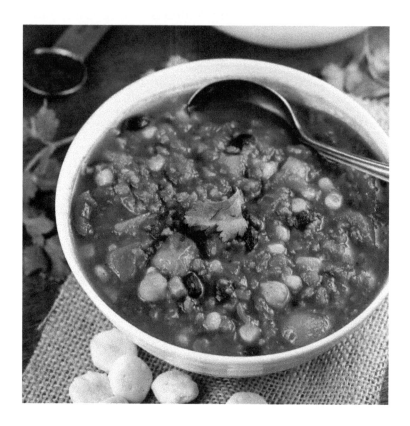

Ingredients

1 red onion, chopped

1 white onion, chopped

8 garlic cloves, minced

1 tsp. shallot, minced

1 15 oz can diced tomatoes

4 cups vegetable broth

1 can water (I use the can of diced tomatoes to grab all the

leftover flavor)

8 oz. dried white beans

1/2 cup vegan Chorizo (Soyrizo), crumbled

2 tablespoons annatto seeds

2 teaspoons cumin

1 tsp. cayenne pepper

1/2 cup uncooked quinoa

1/4 teaspoon sea salt

Directions:

Put all of the ingredients into slow cooker. Cook on low for 8 hours or high for 4 hours. Serve with toppings such as shredded vegan cheese, avocado, green onion and cilantro

Mung Bean and Meatball Chili

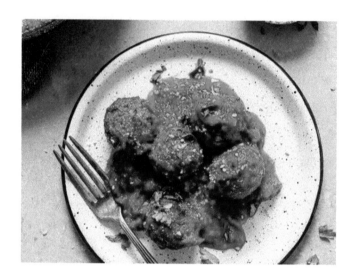

Ingredients

2 red onion, chopped

7 garlic cloves, minced

8 jalapeno peppers, minced

1 tbsp. lemon juice

4 cups vegetable broth

1 can water (I use the can of diced tomatoes to grab all the
leftover flavor)

8 oz. dried mung beans

1/2 cup meatless meatballs, crumbled

2 tablespoons garlic, minced

2 teaspoons chili powder

1 tablespoon Thai chili garlic paste

1/2 cup uncooked black rice

1/4 teaspoon sea salt

Directions:

Put all of the ingredients into slow cooker. Cook on low for 8 hours or high for 4 hours. Serve with toppings such as shredded vegan cheese, avocado, green onion and cilantro

Vegan Burger with White and Black Beans

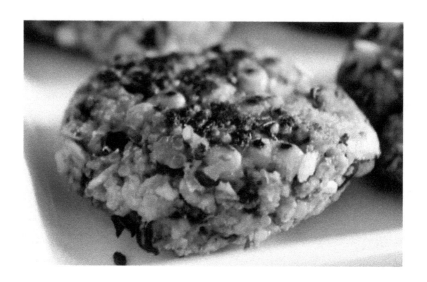

Ingredients

1 red onion, chopped

1 white onion, chopped

8 garlic cloves, minced

1 tsp. shallot, minced

1 15 oz can diced tomatoes

4 cups vegetable broth

1 can water (I use the can of diced tomatoes to grab all the leftover flavor)

8 oz. dried white beans

1/2 cup vegan burger (Brand: Beyond Meat Beyond Burger),

crumbled

2 tablespoons annatto seeds

2 teaspoons cumin

1 tsp. cayenne pepper

1/2 cup uncooked brown rice

1/4 teaspoon sea salt

Directions:

Put all of the ingredients into slow cooker. Cook on low for 8 hours or high for 4 hours. Serve with toppings such as shredded vegan cheese, avocado, green onion and cilantro

Slow Cooked Lima Beans in Pesto Sauce

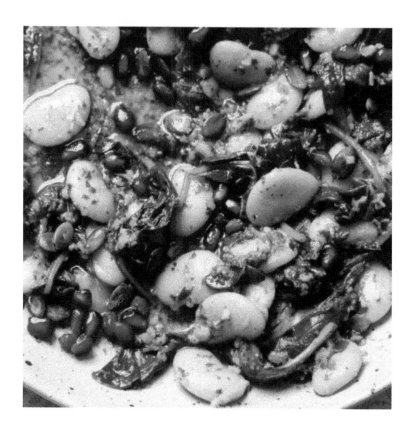

Ingredients

1 red onion, chopped

2 red onions

7 garlic cloves

1 ancho chili, minced

1 tbsp. lime juice

4 cups vegetable broth

1 can water (I use the can of diced tomatoes to grab all the leftover flavor)

8 oz. dried kidney

1 15 oz can Lima Beans

3 tablespoons pesto sauce

1 teaspoons dried basil, coarsely chopped

1 tsp. dried Italian seasoning

1/2 cup uncooked rice

1/4 teaspoon sea salt

Directions:

Put all of the ingredients into slow cooker. Cook on low for 8 hours or high for 4 hours. Serve with toppings such as shredded vegan cheese, avocado, green onion and cilantro

Thai Black Beans Button Mushrooms and Black Rice

Ingredients

1 red onion, chopped

1 yellow onion, chopped

8 garlic cloves, minced

1 tsp. shallot, minced

1 15 oz can diced tomatoes

1 15 oz can button mushrooms

4 cups vegetable broth

1 can water (I use the can of diced tomatoes to grab all the leftover flavor)

8 oz. dried mung beans

1 15 oz can Black Beans

2 tablespoons garlic, minced

2 teaspoons chili powder

1 tablespoon Thai chili garlic paste

1/2 cup uncooked black rice

1/4 teaspoon sea salt

Directions:

Put all of the ingredients into slow cooker. Cook on low for 8 hours or high for 4 hours. Serve with toppings such as shredded vegan cheese, avocado, green onion and cilantro

French Lentils & Black Bean With Red Rice

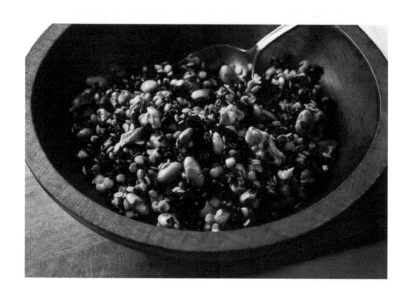

Ingredients

2 red onion, chopped

7 garlic cloves, minced

1 tsp. scallions, minced

1 tbsp. lemon juice

1 15 oz can diced tomatoes

4 cups vegetable broth

1 can water (I use the can of diced tomatoes to grab all the leftover flavor)

8 oz. dried lentils

1 15 oz can Black Beans

2 tablespoons garlic powder

2 teaspoons onion powder

1 tablespoon herbs de Provence

1/2 cup uncooked red rice

1/4 teaspoon sea salt

Directions:

Put all of the ingredients into slow cooker. Cook on low for 8 hours or high for 4 hours. Serve with toppings such as shredded vegan cheese, avocado, green onion and cilantro

Thai Spicy Black Rice and Mung Beans

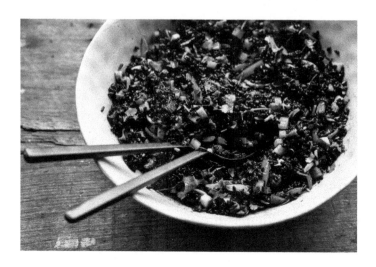

Ingredients

1 red onion, chopped

6 garlic cloves, minced

1 celery stalk, chopped

2 bell peppers, chopped

1 15 oz can diced tomatoes

4 cups vegetable broth

1 can water (I use the can of diced tomatoes to grab all the
leftover flavor)

8 oz. dried mung beans

1 15 oz can Black Beans

2 tablespoons garlic, minced

2 teaspoons chili powder

1 tablespoon Thai chili garlic paste

1/2 cup uncooked black rice

1/4 teaspoon sea salt

Directions:

Put all of the ingredients into slow cooker. Cook on low for 8 hours or high for 4 hours. Serve with toppings such as shredded vegan cheese, avocado, green onion and cilantro

Slow Cooked Tomatoes Rice and Vegan Chorizo

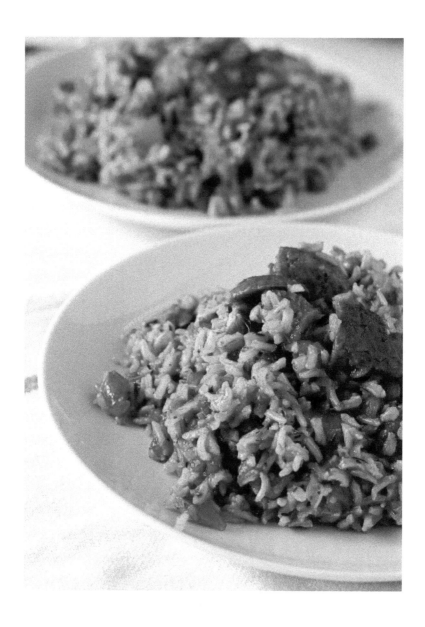

Ingredients

1 red onion, chopped

6 garlic cloves, minced

1 celery stalk, chopped

2 bell peppers, chopped

1 15 oz can diced tomatoes

4 cups vegetable broth

1 can water (I use the can of diced tomatoes to grab all the leftover flavor)

1/2 cup vegan Chorizo (Soyrizo), crumbled

2 tablespoons annatto seeds

2 teaspoons cumin

1 tsp. cayenne pepper

1/2 cup uncooked brown rice

1/4 teaspoon sea salt

Directions:

Put all of the ingredients into slow cooker. Cook on low for 8 hours or high for 4 hours. Serve with toppings such as shredded vegan cheese, avocado, green onion and cilantro

Black Beans and Kidney Beans

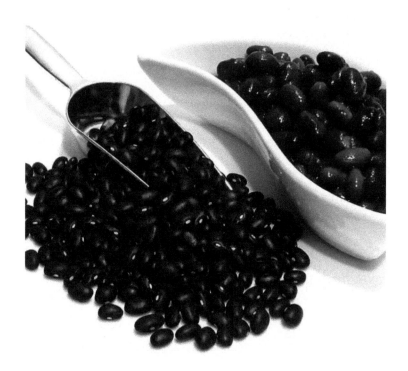

Ingredients

2 red onions

7 garlic cloves

1 ancho chili, minced

1 tbsp. lime juice

4 cups vegetable broth

1 can water (I use the can of diced tomatoes to grab all the leftover flavor)

8 oz. dried kidney beans

1/2 cup vegan Italian sausage, crumbled]

3 tablespoons pesto sauce

1 teaspoons dried basil, coarsely chopped

1 tsp. dried Italian seasoning

1/2 cup uncooked rice

1/4 teaspoon sea salt

Directions:

Put all of the ingredients into slow cooker. Cook on low for 8 hours or high for 4 hours. Serve with toppings such as shredded vegan cheese, avocado, green onion and cilantro

Smoky Quinoa and Meatless Meatballs

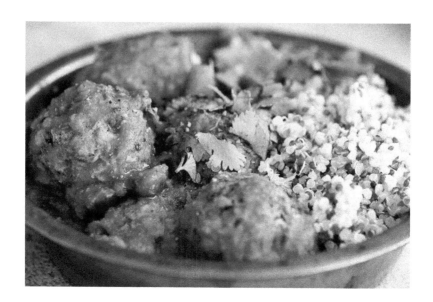

Ingredients

1 red onion, chopped

1 white onion, chopped

8 garlic cloves, minced

1 tsp. shallot, minced

1 15 oz can diced tomatoes

4 cups vegetable broth

1 can water (I use the can of diced tomatoes to grab all the leftover flavor)

1/2 cup meatless meatballs, crumbled

2 tablespoons chili powder

2 teaspoons cumin

1 tablespoon oregano

1/2 cup uncooked quinoa

1/4 teaspoon sea salt

Directions:

Put all of the ingredients into slow cooker. Cook on low for 8 hours or high for 4 hours. Serve with toppings such as shredded vegan cheese, avocado, green onion and cilantro

Black Rice with Enoki Mushrooms

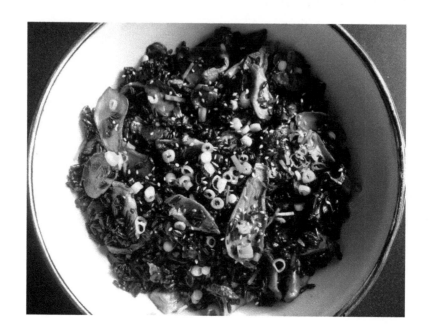

Ingredients

2 red onion, chopped

7 garlic cloves, minced

8 jalapeno peppers, minced

1 tbsp. lemon juice

4 cups vegetable broth

1 can water (I use the can of diced tomatoes to grab all the leftover flavor)

8 oz. dried mung beans

1 15 oz can enoki mushrooms

2 tablespoons garlic, minced

2 teaspoons chili powder

1 tablespoon Thai chili garlic paste

1/2 cup uncooked black rice

1/4 teaspoon sea salt

Directions:

Put all of the ingredients into slow cooker. Cook on low for 8 hours or high for 4 hours. Serve with toppings such as shredded vegan cheese, avocado, green onion and cilantro

Red Rice with Enoki Mushrooms and Tomatoes

Ingredients

1 red onion, chopped

6 garlic cloves, minced

1 celery stalk, chopped

2 bell peppers, chopped

1 15 oz can diced tomatoes

4 cups vegetable broth

1 can water (I use the can of diced tomatoes to grab all the leftover flavor)

8 oz. dried lentils

1 15 oz can enoki mushrooms

2 tablespoons garlic powder

2 teaspoons onion powder

1 tablespoon herbs de Provence

1/2 cup uncooked red rice

1/4 teaspoon sea salt

Directions:

Put all of the ingredients into slow cooker. Cook on low for 8 hours or high for 4 hours. Serve with toppings such as shredded vegan cheese, avocado, green onion and cilantro

Brown Rice with Crimini Mushrooms and Jalapeno Pepper

Ingredients

2 red onion, chopped

7 garlic cloves, minced

8 jalapeno peppers, minced

1 tbsp. lemon juice

4 cups vegetable broth

1 can water (I use the can of diced tomatoes to grab all the leftover flavor)

1 15 oz can crimini mushrooms

2 tablespoons annatto seeds

2 teaspoons cumin

1 tsp. cayenne pepper

1/2 cup uncooked brown rice

1/4 teaspoon sea salt

Directions:

Put all of the ingredients into slow cooker. Cook on low for 8 hours or high for 4 hours. Serve with toppings such as shredded vegan cheese, avocado, green onion and cilantro

Rice with Pesto Sauce and Button Mushrooms

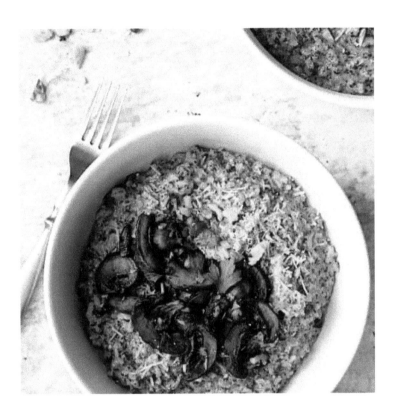

Ingredients

1 red onion, chopped

6 garlic cloves, minced

1 celery stalk, chopped

2 bell peppers, chopped

1 15 oz can diced tomatoes

4 cups vegetable broth

1 can water (I use the can of diced tomatoes to grab all the leftover flavor)

1 15 oz can button mushrooms

3 tablespoons pesto sauce

1 teaspoons dried basil, coarsely chopped

1 tsp. dried Italian seasoning

1/2 cup uncooked rice

1/4 teaspoon sea salt

Directions:

Put all of the ingredients into slow cooker. Cook on low for 8 hours or high for 4 hours. Serve with toppings such as shredded vegan cheese, avocado, green onion and cilantro

Red Rice with Crimini and Button Mushrooms

Ingredients

2 red onion, chopped

7 garlic cloves, minced

1 tsp. scallions, minced

1 tbsp. lemon juice

4 cups vegetable broth

1 can water (I use the can of diced tomatoes to grab all the leftover flavor)

1 cup crimini mushrooms

1 cup button mushrooms

2 tablespoons garlic powder

2 teaspoons onion powder

1 tablespoon herbs de Provence

1/2 cup uncooked red rice

1/4 teaspoon sea salt

Directions:

Put all of the ingredients into slow cooker. Cook on low for 8 hours or high for 4 hours. Serve with toppings such as shredded vegan cheese, avocado, green onion and cilantro

Veggie Pie

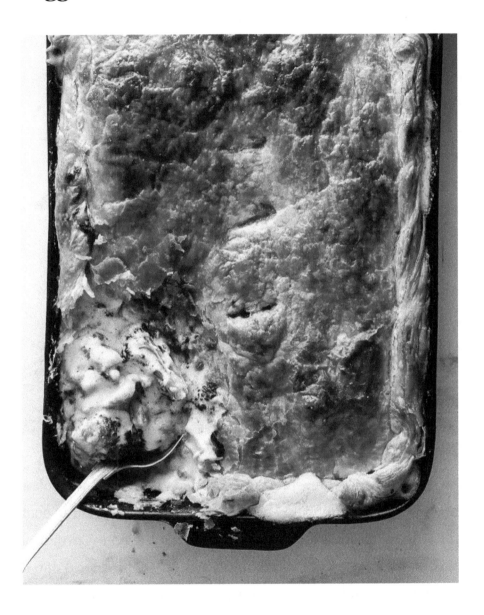

Ingredients

7 cups vegetables chopped into bite sized pieces as needed (I used: brussel sprouts, frozen corn kernels, frozen peas, diced potatoes, baby carrots, and pre-sliced mushrooms)

1/2 cup diced red onion

4 cloves minced garlic

5-6 sprigs fresh thyme leaves removed

1/4 cup flour

2 cups chicken stock

1/4 cup cornstarch

1/4 cup heavy cream

salt and pepper to taste

1 frozen puff pastry sheet thawed

2 tablespoons olive oil

Directions:

Put the 7 cups of vegetables as needed to your slow cooker together with the onion and garlic Combine with the flour to coat well Add the broth until well combined with the flour Cover and cook on high heat for 3 and a half hours or low heat for 6 and a half hours. Combine cornstarch with 1/4 cup water until smooth and add this to the slow cooker. Add the coconut cream, cover, and return slow cooker. Cook on high for 15 minutes or until mixture thickens Transfer to a baking dish and top with the thawed puff pastry sheet. Brush the olive oil over the top of pastry Bake at 400 degrees F for about 10 minutes or until pastry turns golden brown.

Soy Bean and Bell Pepper Soup

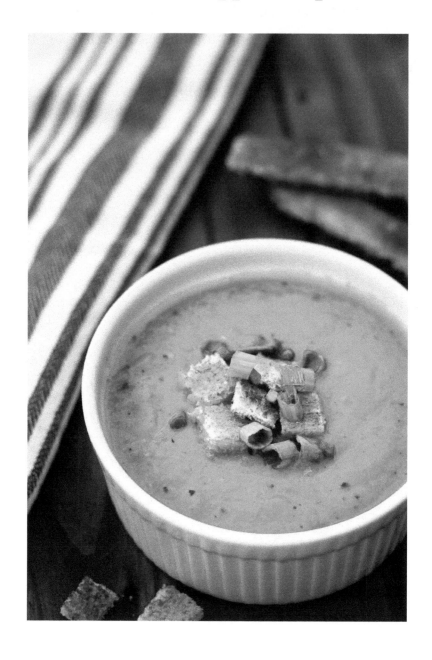

Ingredients

1 pound dry soy beans

4 cups vegetable stock

1 yellow onion, finely chopped

1 green bell pepper, finely chopped

2 jalapeños, seeds removed and finely chopped

1 cup salsa or diced tomatoes

4 teaspoons minced

garlic, about 4 cloves

1 heaping tablespoon chili powder

2 teaspoons ground cumin

2 teaspoons

Sea salt

1 teaspoon ground pepper

1/2 teaspoon ground cayenne pepper (decrease or omit for a milder soup)

1/2 teaspoon smoked paprika

Avocado and cilantro for topping, if desired

Directions:

Completely submerge the beans in water overnight and make sure there's an inch of water over the beans. Drain the beans and rinse. Put the beans, broth, onion, pepper, jalapeños, salsa, garlic, chili powder, cumin, salt, pepper, cayenne, and paprika in a slow cooker. Stir and combine thoroughly. Cook on high heat for 6 hours, until beans are tender. Blend half of the soup until smooth and bring it back to the pot. Top with avocado and cilantro.

Lightning Source UK Ltd.
Milton Keynes UK
UKHW021128110521
383520UK00001B/66